Introduction

Nutrition And Overall Health

Proper nutrition plays a crucial role in maintaining and promoting overall health and well-being. The food we consume provides us with the necessary nutrients, vitamins, and minerals that are essential for the optimal functioning of our bodies. A balanced and nutritious diet not only supports growth and development but also helps prevent various diseases and promotes longevity.

Nutrition is the process of obtaining and utilizing food to fulfill our body's energy requirements and support its physiological functions. It involves the intake of macronutrients, such as carbohydrates, proteins, and fats, as well as micronutrients, including vitamins and minerals. Each of these components has specific roles in the body, and a deficiency or excess of any of them can lead to various health problems.

One of the primary benefits of good nutrition is maintaining a healthy weight. A well-balanced diet, combined with regular physical activity, helps in weight management, preventing obesity and related conditions like diabetes, heart disease, and certain types of cancer. It provides the body with the necessary energy to carry out daily activities, supports muscle growth, and helps regulate metabolism.

Nutrition also plays a vital role in promoting proper growth and development, especially in children and adolescents. During these stages, the body requires an adequate supply of nutrients to support the development of bones, muscles, and organs, as well as cognitive function. Nutritional deficiencies during this period can have long-lasting effects on physical and mental health.

Furthermore, a healthy diet has a significant impact on our immune system. Certain nutrients, such as vitamin C, vitamin D, zinc, and omega-3 fatty acids, play a crucial role in strengthening the immune response, reducing the risk of infections, and aiding in the recovery from illnesses. A well-nourished body can better defend itself against pathogens and maintain optimal immune function.

Proper nutrition is also closely linked to mental health and cognitive function. Research has shown that certain nutrients, including omega-3 fatty acids, B vitamins, and antioxidants, have a positive impact on brain health. They support cognitive function, improve mood, and reduce the risk of mental disorders such as depression and Alzheimer's disease.Nutrition is a fundamental pillar of overall health and well-being. A balanced and nutritious diet provides the body with the necessary nutrients to support growth, development, and optimal functioning.

It helps prevent various diseases, maintain a healthy weight, strengthen the immune system, and support mental health. By prioritizing good nutrition and making informed food choices, we can significantly improve our overall quality of life and longevity.

The Impact of Nutrition on Metabolism

Metabolism is the complex process by which our bodies convert food into energy that fuels various bodily functions. It involves the breakdown of nutrients, their transformation into energy, and the utilization of that energy by cells and organs. Nutrition plays a critical role in metabolism as the macronutrients we consume serve as the building blocks for this energy production.

Macronutrients, namely carbohydrates, proteins, and fats, are the primary sources of energy for the body. Each macronutrient has a unique role in metabolism and provides a different number of calories per gram:

Carbohydrates: Carbohydrates are the body's preferred source of energy. They are broken down into glucose, which is used by cells as fuel. Simple carbohydrates, found in foods like sugar and refined grains, are quickly digested, leading to rapid spikes in blood sugar levels. Complex carbohydrates, found in whole grains, legumes, and vegetables, provide a more sustained release of energy due to their higher fiber content.

Proteins: Proteins are essential for growth, repair, and maintenance of body tissues. During metabolism, proteins are broken down into amino acids, which can be used to build and repair muscles, enzymes, hormones, and other molecules. Unlike carbohydrates and fats, proteins are not the body's preferred source of energy. However, in times of insufficient carbohydrate intake, the body can convert amino acids into glucose through a process called gluconeogenesis.

Fats: Dietary fats provide a concentrated source of energy and play a crucial role in the absorption of fat-soluble vitamins. They are broken down into fatty acids and glycerol during metabolism. Fatty acids can be used as a source of energy, or they can be stored in adipose tissue for future use.

Fat intake also influences hormone regulation and helps maintain healthy cell membranes.

The balance of macronutrients in the diet has a significant impact on metabolism. For example, a high-carbohydrate diet can lead to an increased release of insulin, a hormone that regulates blood sugar levels. Insulin promotes the storage of excess glucose as glycogen in the liver and muscles or as fat in adipose tissue. On the other hand, a diet high in fat and low in carbohydrates can shift the body's primary energy source from glucose to fats, leading to a state of ketosis.

The timing and distribution of macronutrients throughout the day also affect metabolism. For instance, consuming a balanced meal that includes carbohydrates, proteins, and fats can promote a steady release of energy and prevent fluctuations in blood sugar levels. Additionally, regular physical activity and exercise play a vital role in optimizing metabolism by increasing energy expenditure, improving insulin sensitivity, and promoting muscle growth.

Macronutrients serve as the building blocks for metabolism and energy production in the body. Carbohydrates, proteins, and fats are essential for fueling various bodily functions, supporting growth and repair, and maintaining overall health. Understanding the role of macronutrients and making informed dietary choices can help optimize metabolism and contribute to overall well-being.

Carbohydrates

Carbohydrates are one of the three macronutrients and serve as the primary source of energy for the body. They are found in various foods such as grains, fruits, vegetables, legumes, and dairy products. Carbohydrates are broken down into glucose during digestion, which is then used by cells as a fuel source.

Carbohydrates can be classified into two main types: simple carbohydrates and complex carbohydrates. Simple carbohydrates, also known as sugars, include sources like table sugar, honey, and fruit juices. They are quickly digested and provide a rapid but short-lived burst of energy. Complex carbohydrates, on the other hand, are found in foods like whole grains, beans, and vegetables. They contain more fiber and take longer to digest, providing a sustained release of energy.

The body regulates blood sugar levels through the hormone insulin. When we consume carbohydrates, particularly simple carbohydrates, blood sugar levels rise, triggering the release of insulin. Insulin helps transport glucose from the bloodstream into cells for immediate energy use or storage as glycogen in the liver and muscles.

It's important to choose carbohydrates wisely and focus on consuming complex carbohydrates that are high in fiber. These sources provide more sustained energy, help maintain stable blood sugar levels, and support digestive health.

CHAPTER ONE

Proteins

Proteins are crucial for building, repairing, and maintaining tissues in the body. They are made up of amino acids, which are often referred to as the building blocks of proteins. Amino acids are essential for various functions, including the production of enzymes, hormones, antibodies, and structural components like muscles and organs.

There are two types of dietary proteins: complete proteins and incomplete proteins. Complete proteins contain all the essential amino acids that the body cannot produce on its own, and they are found in animal-based sources such as meat, poultry, fish, eggs, and dairy products. Incomplete proteins lack one or more essential amino acids and are commonly found in plant-based sources like legumes, grains, nuts, and seeds. However, by combining different plant-based protein sources throughout the day, it is possible to obtain all the essential amino acids.

Proteins also play a role in metabolism. They have a higher thermic effect compared to carbohydrates and fats, meaning they require more energy to digest, absorb, and metabolize. This can contribute to increased calorie expenditure and can be beneficial for weight management.

Fats

Fats are often misunderstood, but they are an essential part of a healthy diet. Fats provide energy, support cell growth, protect organs, insulate the body, and help absorb fat-soluble vitamins. However, not all fats are created equal.

Saturated fats and trans fats are considered unhealthy fats. Saturated fats are primarily found in animal-based sources such as fatty cuts of meat, full-fat dairy products, and tropical oils like coconut oil. Trans fats are artificially produced through a process called hydrogenation, and they are commonly found in processed and fried foods.

Unsaturated fats, including monounsaturated fats and polyunsaturated fats, are considered healthy fats. They are found in foods such as avocados, nuts, seeds, olive oil, and fatty fish like salmon. These fats can help reduce the risk of heart disease, lower LDL cholesterol levels, and provide essential fatty acids that the body cannot produce on its own.

It's important to moderate fat intake and focus on consuming more unsaturated fats while limiting saturated and trans fats.

Micronutrients

In addition to macronutrients, our bodies also require micronutrients, which include vitamins and minerals. Micronutrients are essential for various biological processes, including energy production, immune function, growth, and development.

Vitamins are organic compounds that are required in small amounts. They are classified into two categories: water-soluble vitamins (such as vitamin C and B vitamins) and fat-soluble vitamins (such as vitamins A, D, E, and K). Each vitamin has specific roles in the body, such as supporting immune function (vitamin C), promoting bone health (vitamin D), and acting as antioxidants (vitamin E).

Minerals are inorganic elements that are necessary for bodily functions. They include calcium, iron, magnesium, zinc, potassium, and many others. Minerals are involved in processes such as bone health, oxygen transport, nerve function, and fluid balance.

A well-balanced diet that includes a variety of whole foods, such as fruits, vegetables, whole grains, lean proteins, and healthy fats, is the best way to ensure an adequate intake of both macronutrients and micronutrients. However, in some cases, dietary supplements may be recommended to address specific deficiencies or medical conditions. It's always advisable to consult a healthcare professional before starting any supplementation.

Understanding the different macronutrients and their impact on the body is crucial for maintaining a healthy diet. Carbohydrates provide energy, proteins are essential for building and repairing tissues, and fats play various roles in the body. Additionally, micronutrients, including vitamins and minerals, are vital for supporting overall health and well-being. By making informed choices and consuming a balanced diet, we can ensure that our bodies receive the necessary nutrients for optimal functioning.

Vitamin A

Vitamin A is a fat-soluble vitamin that plays a crucial role in maintaining healthy vision, promoting immune function, and supporting cell growth and differentiation. It exists in two forms: preformed vitamin A (retinol) found in animal-based foods, and provitamin A carotenoids (beta-carotene) found in plant-based foods.

One of the well-known functions of vitamin A is its role in vision. It is an essential component of rhodopsin, a protein in the retina that allows us to see in low light conditions. Vitamin A deficiency can lead to night blindness and, in severe cases, even total blindness.

Vitamin A also plays a vital role in supporting immune function. It helps maintain the integrity of the skin and mucous membranes, which act as barriers against pathogens. Additionally, it promotes the production and activity of immune cells, such as lymphocytes and macrophages, which are involved in fighting infections.

It's worth noting that while vitamin A is important for health, excessive intake can be harmful. It's essential to follow recommended dietary guidelines and consult with a healthcare professional before taking vitamin A supplements.

Vitamin C

Vitamin C, also known as ascorbic acid, is a water-soluble vitamin with powerful antioxidant properties. It is involved in several critical functions in the body, including collagen synthesis, immune function, and antioxidant protection.

Collagen is a protein that provides structure and strength to various tissues, including skin, bones, tendons, and blood vessels. Vitamin C plays a vital role in the production of collagen, which is essential for wound healing, maintaining healthy skin, and supporting joint health.

Vitamin C is also known for its immune-boosting properties. It supports the production and function of immune cells, such as white blood cells and antibodies, and helps protect against oxidative stress caused by free radicals. Adequate vitamin C intake is important for maintaining a strong immune system and reducing the risk of infections.

Additionally, vitamin C enhances the absorption of iron from plant-based sources, such as beans and leafy greens, when consumed together in the same meal. This is particularly beneficial for individuals following a vegetarian or vegan diet, as iron from plant sources is less easily absorbed compared to iron from animal sources.

Iron

Iron is a mineral that plays a crucial role in various physiological processes, including oxygen transport, energy production, and immune function. It is a component of hemoglobin, the protein in red blood cells that carries oxygen from the lungs to tissues throughout the body.

Iron exists in two forms: heme iron, found in animal-based sources such as red meat and poultry, and non-heme iron, found in plant-based sources like beans, lentils, and spinach. Heme iron is more easily absorbed by the body compared to non-heme iron.

Iron deficiency can lead to iron-deficiency anemia, a condition characterized by decreased production of healthy red blood cells. Symptoms of iron deficiency anemia include fatigue, weakness, pale skin, and impaired cognitive function.

To enhance iron absorption, it is beneficial to consume iron-rich foods along with a source of vitamin C. Vitamin C helps convert non-heme iron into a more absorbable form, increasing

its bioavailability.

CHAPTER TWO

Calcium

Calcium is a mineral that is well-known for its role in maintaining strong bones and teeth. It is the most abundant mineral in the body, with 99% of it stored in the bones and teeth. Calcium also plays a vital role in other bodily functions, including muscle contraction, nerve transmission, and blood clotting.

During periods of growth, such as childhood and adolescence, calcium intake is crucial for the development of strong bones and teeth. However, calcium is important throughout life to maintain bone health and prevent conditions like osteoporosis, which is characterized by weakened and brittle bones.

While dairy products are often associated with calcium, it can also be obtained from other sources such as leafy green vegetables (kale, broccoli), fortified plant-based milks, tofu, and almonds. Adequate vitamin D intake is also important for optimal calcium absorption and utilization.

It's worth noting that calcium absorption can be influenced by other dietary factors, such as excessive sodium, caffeine, and high levels of dietary fiber. It's important to maintain a balanced diet and ensure sufficient calcium intake based on individual needs.

Energy Metabolism

Energy metabolism refers to the complex processes by which our bodies convert food into energy. The energy derived from macronutrients, particularly carbohydrates, proteins, and fats, is utilized to fuel various bodily functions, including cellular activities, organ function, physical activity, and maintaining body temperature.

Understanding our individual caloric needs is essential for maintaining a healthy weight and meeting our energy requirements. Caloric needs vary based on factors such as age, sex, body size, physical activity levels, and overall metabolic rate.

The total energy expenditure (TEE) is the sum of the basal metabolic rate (BMR), which is the energy needed to sustain basic bodily functions at rest, the thermic effect of food (TEF), which is the energy expended during digestion and absorption of food, and the energy expended through physical activity.

To maintain a healthy weight, it's important to balance energy intake (calories consumed through food and beverages) with energy expenditure (calories burned through metabolism and physical activity). Consuming excessive calories can lead to weight gain, while consuming too few calories can lead to weight loss and potential nutrient deficiencies.

It's worth noting that while caloric intake is important, the quality of the diet and the balance of macronutrients also play a significant role in overall health. A balanced diet that includes a variety of nutrient-dense foods is key to supporting energy metabolism and maintaining optimal health.

Vitamins and minerals, such as vitamin A, vitamin C, iron, and calcium, play crucial roles in various bodily functions and are necessary for overall health. Understanding their importance and ensuring adequate intake through a balanced diet can support vision, immune function, collagen production, oxygen transport, bone health, and energy metabolism. Consulting with a healthcare professional or registered dietitian can provide personalized guidance on meeting individual nutrient needs.

Basal Metabolic Rate (BMR) and Total Daily Energy Expenditure (TDEE)

Basal Metabolic Rate (BMR) refers to the amount of energy expended by the body at rest to sustain basic bodily functions, such as breathing, circulating blood, and maintaining body temperature. It represents the largest component of total daily energy expenditure (TDEE), accounting for about 60-75% of the total. Factors affecting BMR are as stated;

Body size and composition: BMR tends to be higher in individuals with more lean muscle mass as muscle tissue is more metabolically active than fat tissue.

Age: BMR tends to decrease with age due to decreases in muscle mass and changes in hormone levels.

Gender: On average, men tend to have a higher BMR compared to women, primarily due to differences in body composition.

Hormonal factors: Hormones, such as thyroid hormones, play a role in regulating metabolism and can affect BMR.

Total Daily Energy Expenditure (TDEE) is the total amount of energy expended by the body in a day, taking into account not only BMR but also physical activity levels and the thermic effect of food (TEF). TEF refers to the energy expended during the digestion, absorption, and storage of nutrients from food.

Factor affecting total daily energy expenditure (TDEE) are as follows;

In addition to BMR and TEF, energy expenditure is influenced by physical activity levels and other factors:

Physical activity: The more active you are, the more energy you expend. Activities such as exercise, walking, and even fidgeting contribute to total energy expenditure.

Non-exercise activity thermogenesis (NEAT): NEAT includes activities like household chores, gardening, and walking that are not specifically exercise-related but still contribute to energy expenditure.

Thermoregulation: Energy expenditure increases in response to extreme temperatures as the body works to maintain its core temperature.

Hormonal factors: Hormones such as adrenaline and cortisol can affect energy expenditure.

CHAPTER THREE

Balancing Energy Intake and Output

To maintain a healthy weight, it's important to balance energy intake (calories consumed) with energy output (calories burned). If energy intake exceeds energy expenditure, weight gain may occur. Conversely, if energy expenditure exceeds energy intake, weight loss may occur.

Monitoring portion sizes, practicing mindful eating, and being aware of hunger and fullness cues can help regulate energy intake. Regular physical activity and exercise can increase energy expenditure, while strength training can help build muscle mass and increase BMR.

Healthy Eating Guidelines

Creating a balanced diet involves incorporating a variety of nutrient-dense foods to meet your nutritional needs. Here are some guidelines:

Macronutrients: Include a balance of carbohydrates, proteins, and fats. Choose whole grains, lean proteins, and healthy fats.

Fruits and vegetables: Aim for a variety of colorful fruits and vegetables, as they provide essential vitamins, minerals, and fiber.

Fiber: Include high-fiber foods like whole grains, legumes, fruits, and vegetables to promote digestion and satiety.

Micronutrients: Ensure adequate intake of vitamins and minerals through a diverse diet or, if necessary, with the guidance of a healthcare professional.

Hydration: Drink plenty of water throughout the day to stay hydrated.

Moderation: Practice moderation with foods high in added sugars, saturated fats, and sodium.

Portion control: Be mindful of portion sizes to avoid excessive calorie intake.

Individual needs: Consider individual factors such as age, sex, activity level, and any specific dietary requirements or restrictions.

It's important to listen to your body's hunger and fullness cues and to consult with a registered dietitian or healthcare professional for personalized guidance on nutrition and creating a balanced diet that meets your specific needs.

The Importance of Portion Control

Portion control is crucial for maintaining a healthy weight and ensuring a balanced intake of nutrients. Here's why portion control is important:

Calorie management: Controlling portion sizes helps manage calorie intake. Consuming more calories than your body needs can lead to weight gain over time. By being mindful of portion sizes, you can better control your calorie intake and support weight management.

Nutrient balance: Proper portion control allows you to create a balanced plate that includes a variety of nutrients. It helps ensure you get adequate amounts of macronutrients (carbohydrates, proteins, and fats) as well as vitamins and minerals.

Hunger and fullness cues: Portion control helps you tune in to your body's hunger and fullness cues. Eating appropriate portions can prevent overeating and promote better satisfaction and satiety after meals.

Tips for practicing portion control include:

- Use smaller plates and bowls to create the illusion of a fuller plate.

- Pay attention to recommended serving sizes on food labels.

- Be mindful of portion sizes when eating out by sharing meals or taking leftovers.

- Use measuring cups, spoons, or a food scale to accurately portion out foods.

The Role of Fiber in Digestive Health

Fiber is an important component of a healthy diet and plays a crucial role in digestive health. Here's why fiber is beneficial:

Promotes regular bowel movements: Fiber adds bulk to the stool and helps prevent constipation by improving the frequency and ease of bowel movements.

Supports gut health: Fiber acts as prebiotic, providing nourishment for beneficial gut bacteria. This promotes a healthy balance of gut microbiota and supports overall gut health.

Helps maintain healthy weight: High-fiber foods are often more filling and can help promote satiety, potentially reducing overall calorie intake and aiding in weight management.

Manages blood sugar levels: Fiber slows down the digestion and absorption of carbohydrates, resulting in a slower and more controlled release of glucose into the bloodstream. This can help stabilize blood sugar levels and prevent spikes and crashes.

To incorporate more fiber into your diet:

- Choose whole grains such as brown rice, quinoa, and whole wheat bread instead of refined grains.

- Include a variety of fruits and vegetables, including those with edible skins or seeds.

- Opt for legumes such as lentils, beans, and chickpeas.

- Snack on nuts, seeds, and high-fiber granola bars.

- Gradually increase your fiber intake to allow your body to adjust.

CHAPTER FOUR

Incorporating Whole Foods for Nutrient Density

Whole foods refer to foods that are in their natural, unprocessed state or have undergone minimal processing. Incorporating whole foods into your diet offers several benefits:

Nutrient density: Whole foods are typically rich in essential nutrients such as vitamins, minerals, antioxidants, and fiber. They provide a wide range of health-promoting compounds that are beneficial for overall well-being.

Lower added sugars and unhealthy fats: Whole foods are generally lower in added sugars, unhealthy fats, and artificial additives that are often found in processed foods. Choosing whole foods helps reduce the intake of these potentially harmful ingredients.

Satiety and portion control: Whole foods are often more filling due to their higher fiber and water content. They can promote satiety, helping you feel satisfied with appropriate portion sizes and potentially reducing the risk of overeating.

Examples of whole foods include fruits, vegetables, whole grains, legumes, nuts, seeds, lean proteins (such as poultry, fish, and tofu), and unprocessed dairy products.

Special Dietary Considerations

Special dietary considerations may arise due to specific health conditions, dietary restrictions, or lifestyle choices. Here are a few examples:

Vegetarian or vegan diets: Vegetarian diets exclude meat and may include dairy and eggs. Vegan diets exclude all animal products. It's important to ensure adequate intake of plant-based protein sources, iron, vitamin B12, omega-3 fatty acids, and other essential nutrients.

Gluten-free diets: Gluten-free diets are essential for individuals with celiac disease or gluten sensitivity. These diets exclude wheat, barley, rye, and their derivatives. It's important to choose gluten-free whole grains, such as quinoa, rice, and gluten-free oats, and to be mindful of hidden sources of gluten in processed foods.

Food allergies or intolerances: Individuals with food allergies or intolerances need to avoid specific allergens or ingredients that trigger adverse reactions. Reading food labels carefully and being aware of potential cross-contamination is crucial.

Medical conditions: Certain medical conditions, such as diabetes, hypertension, or kidney disease, may require dietary modifications. It's important to follow medical advice and work with healthcare professionals or registered dietitians to develop appropriate meal plans.

If you have specific dietary considerations, it's recommended to consult with a registered dietitian or healthcare professional who can provide personalized guidance and support. They can help you navigate your dietary needs while ensuring optimal nutrition and overall well-being.

Vegetarian and Vegan Diets: Meeting Nutritional Needs

Vegetarian and vegan diets can provide adequate nutrition when properly planned to ensure all essential nutrients are obtained. Here are some key considerations:

Protein: Plant-based protein sources include legumes, tofu, tempeh, seitan, quinoa, and soy products. Combining different plant protein sources throughout the day can help ensure all essential amino acids are obtained.

Iron: Plant-based iron sources include legumes, fortified cereals, tofu, tempeh, spinach, and nuts. Iron absorption can be enhanced by consuming vitamin C-rich foods (such as citrus fruits, berries, and bell peppers) alongside iron-rich foods.

Vitamin B12: Vitamin B12 is primarily found in animal products, so supplementation or consuming fortified foods (such as plant-based milks, breakfast cereals, and nutritional yeast) is important for vegans.

Omega-3 fatty acids: Plant-based sources of omega-3 fatty acids include flaxseeds, chia seeds, hemp seeds, walnuts, and algae-based supplements. These can help meet omega-3 requirements, particularly for vegans.

Calcium: Plant-based calcium sources include fortified plant-based milks, tofu made with calcium sulfate, almonds, sesame seeds, and leafy greens like kale and broccoli.

Vitamin D: Vitamin D can be obtained through sunlight exposure, fortified plant-based milks, and supplements. Vegans should ensure adequate sun exposure or consider vitamin D supplementation.

Working with a registered dietitian who specializes in vegetarian and vegan nutrition can provide personalized guidance to meet specific nutrient needs.

Gluten-Free and Dairy-Free Diet

Gluten-free and dairy-free diets are essential for individuals with celiac disease, gluten sensitivity, lactose intolerance, or other medical conditions. Here are some tips for navigating these dietary restrictions:

Gluten-free: Choose naturally gluten-free whole grains like rice, quinoa, corn, and gluten-free oats. Use gluten-free flours (such as almond flour, coconut flour, or rice flour) for baking. Be mindful of cross-contamination in food preparation and carefully read food labels to avoid hidden sources of gluten.

Dairy-free: Replace dairy milk with plant-based alternatives like almond, soy, coconut, or oat milk. Look for dairy-free alternatives to cheese, yogurt, and ice cream made from nuts, seeds, or soy. Fortified plant-based milks can provide nutrients like calcium and vitamin D typically obtained from dairy.

Nutrient considerations: Pay attention to nutrient intake, particularly calcium, vitamin D, vitamin B12, and zinc. Include plant-based sources of these nutrients or consider fortified foods and supplements as necessary.

CHAPTER FIVE

Managing Food Allergies and Intolerances

Individuals with food allergies or intolerances must avoid specific allergens or ingredients that trigger adverse reactions. Here are some tips for managing food allergies and intolerances:

Read food labels: Carefully read food labels to identify potential allergens or ingredients that may cause adverse reactions.

Cross-contamination: Be aware of potential cross-contamination in food preparation, both at home and when dining out. This may involve separate utensils, cookware, and food preparation areas.

Seek alternatives: Find suitable alternatives for allergenic ingredients. For example, use allergen-free flours (like chickpea flour or rice flour) for baking, replace dairy with non-dairy alternatives, and explore creative ingredient substitutions.

Work with healthcare professionals: Consult with healthcare professionals, such as allergists or registered dietitians, who can provide guidance and support for managing specific allergies or intolerances.

Nutrition for Different Life Stages

Nutritional needs vary at different life stages, including childhood, adolescence, adulthood, pregnancy, and older adulthood. Here are some key considerations:

Childhood and adolescence: Proper nutrition is crucial for growth and development. Ensure a balanced diet with adequate calories, proteins, healthy fats, vitamins, and minerals. Pay attention to nutrients like calcium, iron, and vitamin D, which are important during these stages.

Pregnancy: Adequate nutrition is vital during pregnancy to support the health of both the mother and the developing baby. Focus on nutrient-dense foods, including folate-rich foods, iron, calcium, omega-3 fatty acids, and sufficient calories. Prenatal supplements may be recommended.

Adulthood: Maintain a balanced diet that meets energy needs and supports overall health. Focus on nutrient-dense foods and incorporate regular physical activity.

Older adulthood: Nutritional needs may change with age. Ensure sufficient intake of nutrients like calcium, vitamin D, vitamin B12, and fiber. Adequate hydration, regular physical activity, and maintaining social connections are also important.

Consulting with a registered dietitian can provide personalized guidance tailored to specific life stages and individual needs. They can help create meal plans and address any specific concerns or requirements.

Prenatal Nutrition

Prenatal nutrition is crucial for supporting a healthy pregnancy and the growth and development of the baby. Here are key considerations:

Folate: Adequate folate intake is important for the prevention of neural tube defects in the developing fetus. Include folate-rich foods such as leafy greens, legumes, fortified cereals, and prenatal supplements.

Iron: Iron needs increase during pregnancy to support the production of red blood cells and prevent iron-deficiency anemia. Include iron-rich foods like lean meats, fortified cereals, beans, and leafy greens. Iron supplementation may be recommended.

Calcium and vitamin D: Calcium is essential for the development of the baby's bones and teeth, while vitamin D supports calcium absorption. Include dairy products or fortified plant-based milks and spend time outdoors for natural vitamin D synthesis.

Omega-3 fatty acids: Omega-3 fatty acids, particularly DHA, are important for fetal brain and eye development. Include fatty fish (low in mercury) or consider algae-based supplements if following a vegetarian or vegan diet.

Hydration: Stay hydrated by drinking plenty of water throughout the day.

Consult with a healthcare professional for personalized advice on prenatal nutrition and appropriate supplementation.

Childhood Nutrition

Childhood nutrition plays a critical role in growth, development, and overall health. Here are some considerations:

Balanced meals: Provide a variety of nutrient-dense foods from all food groups, including fruits, vegetables, whole grains, lean proteins, and dairy products or plant-based alternatives.

Essential nutrients: Ensure adequate intake of nutrients like calcium, iron, vitamin D, and omega-3 fatty acids. Encourage consumption of dairy products, fortified plant-based milks, lean meats, fish, eggs, and plant-based sources.

Limit added sugars and processed foods: Minimize intake of sugary beverages, snacks, and processed foods. Encourage whole, unprocessed foods whenever possible.

Hydration: Promote regular water intake throughout the day.

Role modeling and family meals: Set a positive example by practicing healthy eating habits and enjoying regular family meals together.

Education and involvement: Teach children about the importance of healthy eating, involve them in meal planning and preparation, and encourage them to make nutritious choices.

Consult with a registered dietitian or pediatrician for personalized guidance on childhood nutrition.

CHAPTER SIX

Nutrition for Aging Gracefully

As we age, nutrition plays a crucial role in maintaining health and well-being. Here are some considerations for nutrition in older adulthood:

Nutrient-dense foods: Focus on nutrient-dense options to meet nutritional needs while managing calorie intake. Include fruits, vegetables, whole grains, lean proteins, low-fat dairy or plant-based alternatives, and healthy fats.

Fiber: Adequate fiber intake supports digestive health. Include whole grains, fruits, vegetables, legumes, and nuts in the diet.

Hydration: Pay attention to hydration, as older adults may have a reduced sense of thirst. Drink water regularly and consume hydrating foods like fruits and vegetables.

Calcium and vitamin D: Maintain bone health by including calcium-rich foods and ensuring adequate vitamin D through sunlight exposure or supplementation.

Protein: Aim for sufficient protein intake to support muscle strength and prevent muscle loss. Include lean meats, fish, poultry, dairy products or plant-based alternatives, legumes, and nuts.

Limit added sugars and sodium: Minimize intake of sugary snacks, beverages, and processed foods, and monitor sodium intake to support heart health.

Consult with a healthcare professional or registered dietitian for personalized guidance on nutrition for aging gracefully.

Sports Nutrition

Sports nutrition is essential for athletes to optimize performance, support recovery, and maintain overall health. Here are some key considerations:

Energy needs: Determine individual energy requirements based on activity level, goals, and body composition. Balance calorie intake with expenditure to support energy needs.

Macronutrients: Ensure sufficient intake of carbohydrates for fueling exercise, protein for muscle repair and recovery, and healthy fats for energy and hormone regulation.

Timing of meals and snacks: Consume meals and snacks strategically to provide fuel before, during, and after exercise. Pre-workout meals should include carbohydrates and a moderate amount of protein, while post-workout meals should focus on replenishing glycogen stores and providing protein for muscle repair.

Hydration: Stay hydrated before, during, and after exercise. Monitor fluid intake and consider electrolyte replacement for prolonged or intense exercise.

Sports-specific considerations: Different sports may have unique nutritional requirements. Seek guidance from sports dietitian who can provide personalized advice based on specific athletic goals and needs.

Supplements: Use caution with supplements and consult a sports dietitian or healthcare professional before incorporating any supplements into your regimen.

Sports nutrition should be tailored to individual needs, taking into account specific sport requirements, training intensity, and personal goals. Working with a sports dietitian can provide personalized guidance for optimal performance.

Pre- and Post-Workout Nutrition Strategies

Pre- and post-workout nutrition plays a vital role in optimizing performance, supporting energy levels, and promoting recovery. Here are some strategies:

Pre-workout:

Carbohydrates: Consume a small meal or snack that includes carbohydrates to provide energy for the workout. Opt for easily digestible options such as fruits, whole grains, or a small portion of complex carbohydrates.

Protein: Include a moderate amount of protein to support muscle repair and provide amino acids for muscle building. Options like Greek yogurt, a protein shake, or a small portion of lean protein can be beneficial.

Timing: Eat a pre-workout meal or snack 1-3 hours before exercising to allow for digestion. Experiment to find the timing that works best for your body and workout routine.

Post-workout:

Carbohydrates: Consume carbohydrates to replenish glycogen stores and support recovery. Opt for fast-digesting carbohydrates like fruits, rice cakes, or a sports drink immediately after exercise.

Protein: Include a source of protein to support muscle repair and synthesis. Options like lean meats, poultry, fish, eggs, dairy products or plant-based alternatives, or protein shakes can be beneficial.

Timing: Consume a post-workout meal or snack within 30-60 minutes after exercise to take advantage of the post-workout recovery window when your body is most receptive to nutrient uptake.

Hydration

Hydration is crucial for maintaining performance and preventing dehydration during exercise. Here are some hydration strategies:

Fluid intake: Drink fluids before, during, and after exercise to maintain hydration. Water is generally sufficient for workouts of moderate intensity and duration.

Electrolytes: For prolonged or intense exercise, consider consuming fluids or sports drinks that contain electrolytes to replace those lost through sweat. Electrolytes help maintain fluid balance and support proper muscle and nerve function.

Individual needs: Hydration needs vary depending on factors such as intensity, duration, weather conditions, and individual sweat rates. Monitor your body's hydration cues and adjust fluid intake accordingly.

Pre-hydration: Start exercise well-hydrated by drinking fluids in the hours leading up to your workout. This can help ensure adequate hydration status before you begin.

Optimizing Recovery and Muscle Growth

Recovery nutrition is essential for repairing muscles, replenishing energy stores, and promoting adaptation and growth. Consider the following strategies:

Protein: Consume an adequate amount of protein post-workout to support muscle repair and growth. Aim for 20-30 grams of high-quality protein from sources such as lean meats, poultry, fish, dairy products or plant-based alternatives, eggs, or protein shakes.

Carbohydrates: Include carbohydrates in your post-workout meal or snack to replenish glycogen stores and support recovery. Opt for a combination of fast-digesting carbohydrates and slower-digesting complex carbohydrates.

Nutrient timing: Consume a balanced meal or snack within the post-workout recovery window (30-60 minutes) to maximize nutrient uptake and support optimal recovery.

Hydration: Rehydrate by drinking fluids after exercise to replace any fluid losses. Water is typically sufficient for moderate-intensity workouts, but sports drinks with electrolytes may be beneficial for more intense or prolonged exercise.

Rest and sleep: Ensure sufficient rest and quality sleep to support recovery and muscle growth.

Healthy Weight Management

Maintaining a healthy weight involves a combination of balanced nutrition, regular physical activity, and lifestyle factors. Consider the following strategies:

Caloric balance: Find the right balance between energy intake and expenditure to support weight management. Create a moderate calorie deficit through a combination of diet and exercise for gradual and sustainable weight loss.

Portion control: Practice portion control to manage calorie intake and avoid overeating. Be mindful of portion sizes and listen to your body's hunger and fullness cues.

Balanced diet: Focus on a balanced diet that includes nutrient-dense foods from all food groups. Emphasize fruits, vegetables, whole grains, lean proteins, and healthy fats. Limit added sugars, saturated fats, and processed foods.

Regular physical activity: Incorporate a combination of aerobic exercise, strength training, and flexibility exercises into your routine. Aim for at least 150 minutes of moderate-intensity aerobic activity per week, along with muscle-strengthening activities.

Mindful eating: Practice mindful eating by paying attention to your food choices, eating slowly, and savoring each bite. This can help prevent overeating and improve the overall eating experience.

Lifestyle factors: Prioritize quality sleep, manage stress levels, and cultivate a supportive environment to promote overall well-being and healthy weight management.

Consult with a registered dietitian or healthcare professional for personalized guidance and support on weight management strategies that are appropriate for your individual needs and goals.

CHAPTER SEVEN

Understanding Body Mass Index (BMI)

Body Mass Index (BMI) is a widely used tool to assess body weight status and estimate the level of body fat. It is calculated by dividing a person's weight in kilograms by the square of their height in meters. The formula for BMI is:

$$BMI = weight (kg) / height^2 (m^2)$$

The resulting BMI value is then classified into different categories:

- Underweight: BMI less than 18.5

- Normal weight: BMI 18.5 to 24.9

- Overweight: BMI 25 to 29.9

- Obesity: BMI 30 or higher

While BMI can be a useful screening tool for population studies, it has limitations when assessing individuals. It does not account for variations in body composition, such as muscle mass, and does not provide information about the distribution of body fat. Therefore, it's important to interpret BMI alongside other factors such as waist circumference, body composition analysis, and overall health markers.

The Role of Diet and Exercise in Weight Loss

Diet and exercise are key components in achieving and maintaining weight loss. Here's how they contribute:

Diet: A healthy, balanced diet is crucial for weight loss. It involves consuming nutrient-dense foods in appropriate portion sizes while reducing calorie intake. Focus on whole foods, including fruits, vegetables, lean proteins, whole grains, and healthy fats. Limit added sugars, saturated fats, and processed foods. Consider working with a registered dietitian for personalized guidance.

Exercise: Regular physical activity helps burn calories, increase metabolism, and improve overall fitness. Aim for a combination of cardiovascular exercise (such as walking, jogging, cycling) and strength training to build lean muscle mass. Consult with a fitness professional to develop an exercise plan that suits your abilities and goals.

Caloric balance: Weight loss occurs when there is a calorie deficit, meaning you consume fewer calories than you burn. This can be achieved through a combination of diet and exercise. It's important to create a moderate calorie deficit and avoid extreme diets or overly restrictive eating patterns.

Establishing Healthy Habits for Long-Term Success

Sustainable weight loss and long-term success require establishing healthy habits. Here are some tips:

Set realistic goals: Set achievable and measurable goals that align with your long-term vision. Break them down into smaller, manageable steps to maintain motivation and track progress.

Make gradual changes: Focus on making small, sustainable changes to your eating and exercise habits. This allows for easier adjustment and long-lasting adherence.

Adopt a balanced approach: Avoid extreme diets or drastic measures. Instead, aim for a balanced and varied diet that includes all food groups. Incorporate enjoyable physical activities into your routine to maintain engagement.

Practice portion control: Be mindful of portion sizes to manage calorie intake.

Use smaller plates and bowls, read food labels for serving sizes, and practice listening to your body's hunger and fullness cues.

Meal planning and preparation: Plan and prepare meals and snacks in advance to support healthy choices and avoid impulsive, unhealthy options. This can help with portion control and nutrient-dense meals.

Regular physical activity: Make physical activity a regular part of your routine. Find activities you enjoy and make them a priority. Aim for consistency rather than perfection.

Nutrition Misconceptions and Fads

In the realm of nutrition, it's important to be critical and discerning about misinformation and fad diets. Here are some tips:

Rely on evidence-based information: Seek information from reputable sources such as registered dietitians, scientific journals, and well-established health organizations. Be cautious of misinformation found on social media or from unqualified sources.

Individualization: Remember that nutrition needs can vary based on individual factors such as age, sex, activity level, health conditions, and personal preferences. What works for one person may not work for another.

Balance and moderation: Avoid extremes and embrace a balanced approach to nutrition. Restrictive diets or eliminating entire food groups can lead to nutrient deficiencies and an unhealthy relationship with food. Emphasize variety, moderation, and enjoyment in eating.

Long-term sustainability: Look for eating patterns and lifestyle habits that can be sustained in the long term. Quick fixes or short-term diets are rarely effective or sustainable for lasting weight loss and overall health.

Consult professionals: If you have specific nutrition concerns or require personalized guidance, consult with a registered dietitian or healthcare professional. They can provide evidence-based recommendations tailored to your needs.

By focusing on established principles of nutrition, adopting a balanced approach, and seeking guidance from qualified professionals, you can navigate the world of nutrition and make informed decisions for your health and weight management journey.

CHAPTER EIGHT

Assessing the Validity of Popular Diets

When evaluating popular diets, it's important to consider their validity and suitability for your individual needs. Here are some factors to consider:

Scientific evidence: Look for diets that are supported by scientific research and have been studied for their safety and effectiveness. Pay attention to the quality and quantity of research conducted on the diet.

Balanced approach: Consider whether the diet promotes a balanced intake of macronutrients, vitamins, and minerals. Avoid extreme diets that eliminate entire food groups or severely restrict calorie intake, as they may lead to nutrient deficiencies or imbalances.

Long-term sustainability: Assess whether the diet can be maintained in the long term. Sustainable diets are those that can be integrated into a person's lifestyle and support lifelong healthy eating habits.

Individual needs: Consider your own health goals, preferences, and any specific dietary requirements or restrictions. The best diet for one person may not be suitable for another. Consulting with a registered dietitian can provide personalized guidance.

The Power of Small Changes for Big Impact

Small changes in eating habits and lifestyle can have a significant impact on overall health and well-being. Here are some examples:

Portion control: Practice mindful eating and be aware of portion sizes. Use smaller plates, bowls, and utensils to help control portion sizes and avoid overeating.

Balanced meals: Aim for balanced meals that include a variety of nutrient-dense foods. Fill half your plate with vegetables, one-quarter with lean protein, and one-quarter with whole grains or starchy vegetables.

Snack smartly: Choose healthy snacks like fruits, vegetables with hummus, or a handful of nuts instead of sugary or processed snacks. This can help reduce calorie intake and provide essential nutrients.

Hydration: Stay hydrated by drinking water throughout the day. Carry a reusable water bottle with you as a reminder to drink regularly.

Physical activity: Incorporate physical activity into your daily routine. Take the stairs instead of the elevator, go for a walk during lunch breaks, or find activities you enjoy that get you moving.

Sustaining Lifelong Nutrition Habits

Sustaining lifelong nutrition habits is key to long-term health and well-being. Here are some strategies to support lasting changes:

Mindset shift: Embrace a positive and flexible mindset towards food and nutrition. Focus on nourishing your body rather than restrictive or negative approaches to eating.

Set realistic goals: Set achievable, realistic goals that align with your long-term vision. Break them down into smaller steps and celebrate each milestone along the way.

Accountability and support: Seek support from family, friends, or a community of like-minded individuals who share similar health goals. This can provide motivation, accountability, and a sense of belonging.

Education and learning: Stay informed about nutrition by reading reputable sources, attending workshops or seminars, and consulting with registered dietitians. Continually expand your knowledge and adapt your habits accordingly.

Flexibility and adaptability: Recognize that life circumstances and priorities may change over time. Be open to adjusting your nutrition habits to fit your current needs and circumstances.

Self-care and balance: Prioritize self-care and find a balance that works for you. This includes taking time for relaxation, managing stress, getting adequate sleep, and finding joy in the foods you eat.

Remember that sustainable nutrition habits are built over time. Focus on progress rather than perfection, and be patient and kind to yourself as you work towards long-lasting changes.

Conclusion

Nutrition plays a critical role in overall health and well-being. By understanding the importance of nutrition, we can make informed choices to support our bodies and promote optimal health. A nutrient-rich lifestyle involves consuming a balanced diet that includes a variety of fruits, vegetables, whole grains, lean proteins, and healthy fats.

It also requires incorporating regular physical activity, staying hydrated, and adopting healthy habits that can be sustained in the long term.

It is important to debunk common nutrition myths, assess the validity of popular diets based on scientific evidence and individual needs, and understand the power of small changes for significant impact. By establishing healthy habits and making gradual adjustments to our eating and lifestyle patterns, we can set ourselves up for success and maintain lifelong nutrition practices.

THE END

THE END